New Year, New Adventures

The Best Wellness Retreats for 2025

OLIVIA HARPER

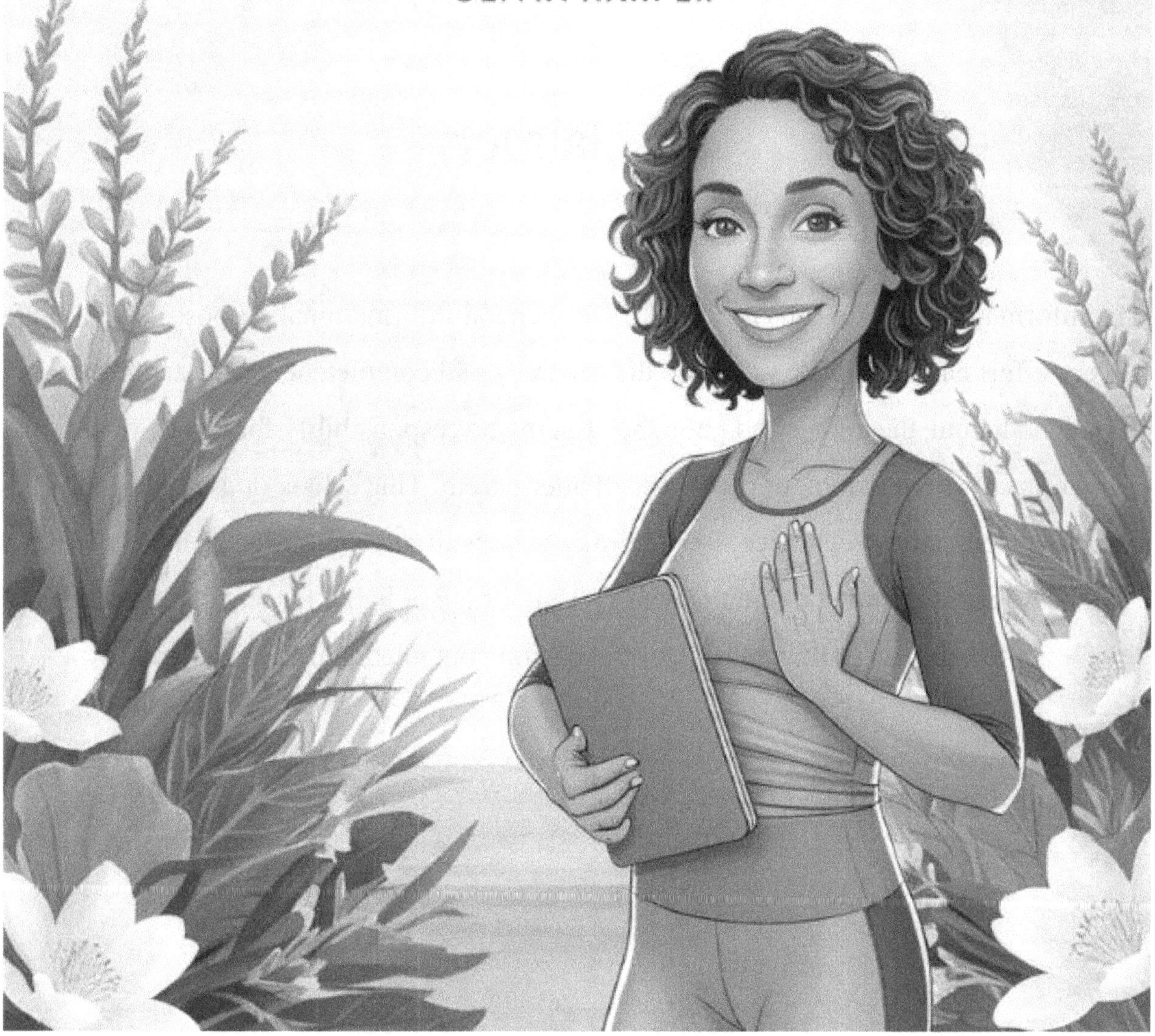

Copyright © 2024 by Olivia Harper

Disclaimer:

The information provided in this eBook is for general informational purposes only. While every effort has been made to ensure the accuracy and completeness of the information contained herein, the author and publisher assume no responsibility for errors, omissions, or contrary interpretation of the subject matter herein. This eBook does not constitute legal, financial, or travel advice. Readers should consult relevant professionals or experts for specific advice suited to their needs. The author is not liable for any damages arising from the use or misuse of the information contained in this publication.

About the Author

Olivia Harper is a wellness enthusiast, travel expert, and author of several travel guides focused on immersive and transformative experiences. With over a decade of experience in wellness tourism, she has traveled extensively to discover retreats that promote healing, mindfulness, and well-being. Olivia is passionate about helping others lead healthier, more mindful lives by exploring new cultures and integrating wellness practices into everyday living. When she's not writing, Olivia can be found practicing yoga, hiking, or planning her next wellness journey.

Table of Contents

Introduction

New Year, New Adventures: The Best Wellness Retreats for 2025

As the clock strikes midnight and the new year begins, many of us are filled with a sense of hope and renewal. There's something about turning the page to a fresh calendar year that inspires change, transformation, and new adventures. Whether you're aiming to improve your physical health, recharge mentally, or embark on a spiritual journey, 2025 is the perfect time to prioritize wellness and embark on life-changing travel experiences.

Wellness retreats offer a unique opportunity to step away from the stresses of daily life, reconnect with yourself, and cultivate healthy habits that last well beyond your time away. In recent years, the wellness travel industry has exploded in popularity, offering a wide array of retreats designed to nourish the mind, body, and soul. From tranquil yoga sanctuaries in Bali to cutting-edge wellness centers in the United States, there's a retreat for everyone, regardless of budget, interest, or location.

This guide is your ticket to discovering the top wellness retreats for 2025, designed to help you rejuvenate, heal, and explore new horizons. In this introduction, we'll dive into the essence of wellness retreats, why they matter now more than ever, and practical tips for making the most of your wellness journey this year.

Why Wellness Travel Matters in 2025

After a few tumultuous years, people across the globe are recognizing the importance of health, both mental and physical, as the foundation of a fulfilling life. Wellness travel is more than a passing trend—it's a conscious choice to prioritize self-care and personal growth in an environment designed to support your well-being. The beauty of wellness retreats is that they offer a holistic approach to rejuvenation, combining physical activities, mental clarity practices, nutritional balance, and often, spiritual guidance.

In 2025, the landscape of wellness retreats continues to evolve, reflecting a deep desire for connection, healing, and sustainability. You'll find a strong emphasis on digital detoxes—where guests are encouraged (or required) to disconnect from the constant buzz of technology. Eco-friendly retreats focused on sustainability and integrating local cultures are also on the rise, as travelers seek experiences that not only benefit their well-being but also have a positive impact on the environment and local communities.

What to Expect from This Guide

This guide is carefully crafted to provide you with the best options for wellness retreats in 2025. Whether you're looking for a transformative yoga retreat in the mountains, a luxurious spa escape, or a remote digital detox in the desert, you'll find a diverse range of experiences that cater to various needs and desires.

Here's a sneak peek of what's to come:

- **Wellness Retreat Trends for 2025**: Discover the hottest trends in wellness travel, from immersive cultural experiences to retreats that use cutting-edge technology.
- **Top Wellness Retreats by Region**: Explore top retreats across North America, Europe, Asia, and beyond, each offering unique settings, treatments, and approaches to well-being.
- **Budgeting for Your Wellness Retreat**: Whether you're on a tight budget or looking for a luxury experience, we'll show you how to find the right retreat without breaking the bank.

- **Practical Tips for a Successful Retreat**: Learn how to set intentions, pack the essentials, and make the most of your retreat experience for lasting results.

The Essence of Wellness Retreats

A wellness retreat is much more than a simple vacation. While traditional holidays often focus on sightseeing and relaxation, wellness retreats are purposefully designed to offer an immersive experience that promotes healing, personal growth, and overall well-being. Whether you're drawn to retreats centered around yoga, meditation, fitness, detox, or spa treatments, they share a common goal: to help you disconnect from everyday life and reconnect with your true self.

Key Benefits of Wellness Retreats:

1. **Mental Rejuvenation**: Most of us live fast-paced lives, juggling work, family, and a never-ending stream of responsibilities. Wellness retreats offer a peaceful environment to unwind, practice mindfulness, and rejuvenate your mental clarity. Whether through meditation, nature walks, or silent retreats, you'll return home with a clearer, calmer mind.

2. **Physical Health**: Many wellness retreats integrate physical activities into their programs. Yoga retreats, for instance, offer daily practice to improve flexibility, strength, and balance. Fitness-focused retreats may include personal training, hiking, and group workouts to kickstart a healthier lifestyle.

3. **Emotional Healing**: Life's challenges can take a toll on our emotional well-being. Wellness retreats often provide tools such as journaling, breathwork, or counseling sessions to help guests heal emotionally, reflect on their lives, and build healthier coping mechanisms.

4. **Spiritual Growth**: For those seeking a deeper connection to their inner selves, spiritual retreats offer opportunities for personal exploration. Whether it's

practicing yoga in a serene mountain setting, participating in guided meditation, or engaging in holistic therapies like Reiki or sound healing, spiritual growth is often a key part of the retreat experience.

Why 2025 is the Perfect Year for a Wellness Retreat

The start of a new year always feels like the ideal time to invest in self-care and set new intentions. In 2025, global wellness travel is not only more accessible but also more diverse than ever before. As people seek meaning and fulfillment beyond material success, they are increasingly turning to wellness retreats as a way to reset and recharge.

With more options than ever, 2025 offers:

- **Diverse Retreat Locations**: From tropical beaches to serene forests, wellness retreats are now offered in stunning locations all over the world. Choose a retreat based on your ideal environment—whether it's the tranquility of the mountains, the healing power of the ocean, or the serenity of the desert.
- **Focus on Sustainability**: Travelers are increasingly looking for eco-conscious retreats that align with their values. Many wellness centers have adopted sustainable practices, such as using local, organic foods and building eco-friendly accommodations.
- **Customizable Experiences**: Many retreats now offer flexible schedules, allowing you to personalize your experience based on your wellness goals. Whether you're there to focus on fitness, mental clarity, or simply relax, you can tailor your retreat to fit your needs.

Practical Tips for Choosing a Wellness Retreat in 2025

When selecting a wellness retreat, it's essential to consider what you hope to achieve from the experience. Here are a few tips to help you make the best choice:

1. **Set Clear Intentions**: Before booking your retreat, ask yourself what you want to gain. Are you looking for physical healing, emotional balance, or spiritual growth? Defining your goals will help you choose a retreat that aligns with your desires.

2. **Research the Location**: Each retreat offers a different environment that can greatly impact your experience. If you need complete solitude, consider a remote location. If you thrive in vibrant cultures, a retreat that incorporates local customs might be more suitable.

3. **Check Reviews and Testimonials**: Wellness retreats can be a significant investment, so make sure to read reviews and testimonials from previous guests. This can give you insight into the quality of the accommodations, treatments, and overall experience.

4. **Consider the Program's Structure**: Some retreats follow a highly structured schedule, while others offer a more relaxed, go-at-your-own-pace approach. Choose a structure that feels comfortable for you, especially if this is your first wellness retreat.

5. **Mind Your Budget**: Wellness retreats can range from affordable to ultra-luxurious. Be mindful of additional costs, such as flights, extra services, or meals. Look for all-inclusive retreats or those that fit your budget without compromising on the experience.

Chapter 1:

The Essence of Wellness Retreats

In today's fast-paced world, the demands of work, relationships, and daily responsibilities can take a toll on our mental, physical, and emotional well-being. It's no surprise that people are increasingly seeking ways to escape, rejuvenate, and reconnect with themselves. Enter wellness retreats—a growing trend that promises holistic healing through mindfulness, fitness, and self-care practices.

Wellness retreats are more than just vacations; they're immersive experiences designed to nurture your mind, body, and spirit. This chapter will explore what defines a wellness retreat, the types of retreats available, their benefits, and how to choose the right one for you. By the end of this chapter, you'll have a clear understanding of why wellness retreats are one of the best investments you can make for yourself in 2025.

What Defines a Wellness Retreat?

A wellness retreat is a getaway specifically designed to promote physical, mental, and spiritual well-being. Unlike traditional vacations that may focus solely on relaxation or adventure, wellness retreats offer structured programs that combine fitness, mindfulness, nutrition, and self-discovery. They often take place in tranquil environments, such as mountains, beaches, or forests, to provide a peaceful backdrop for reflection and growth.

Wellness retreats typically include a schedule of activities, such as yoga, meditation, fitness classes, spa treatments, and workshops on topics like healthy living or personal development. These activities are meant to help participants disconnect from the stresses of daily life and reconnect with themselves in a meaningful way.

Key Features of Wellness Retreats:

1. **Holistic Approach:** Focus on healing the body, mind, and spirit as a whole.
2. **Expert Guidance:** Led by experienced instructors, therapists, or wellness professionals.
3. **Tranquil Environment:** Set in serene locations, free from distractions of everyday life.
4. **Structured Schedule:** A balanced combination of physical activities, relaxation, and personal growth.
5. **Focus on Rejuvenation:** Aimed at restoring balance and promoting long-term well-being.

Types of Wellness Retreats

The beauty of wellness retreats is their diversity. Whether you want to detox, reduce stress, improve your fitness, or explore your spiritual side, there's a retreat for you. Below are some of the most popular types of wellness retreats:

1. **Yoga Retreats:**

   Yoga retreats focus on physical postures (asanas), breathing techniques (pranayama), and meditation to promote balance, flexibility, and mental clarity. They are ideal for those seeking a deeper connection between their mind and body. Many yoga retreats offer beginner to advanced programs, so you don't need to be a seasoned yogi to attend.

   Example: Ananda in the Himalayas, India, combines yoga and Ayurveda practices to help guests restore their natural balance.

2. **Meditation and Mindfulness Retreats:**

   These retreats emphasize mental clarity and emotional healing through meditation and mindfulness practices. They help participants cultivate inner peace, reduce stress, and improve concentration. Many retreats offer silent meditation, where participants refrain from speaking for several days to deepen their mindfulness practice.

Example: Vipassana Meditation Retreats are held worldwide and offer a 10-day silent retreat to focus on mindfulness.

3. **Detox and Cleansing Retreats:**

Designed to eliminate toxins from the body, detox retreats focus on clean eating, juicing, fasting, and natural therapies like colon hydrotherapy. They are ideal for people looking to reset their digestive system, boost their immune system, and kick-start a healthier lifestyle.

Example: The Detox Barn in the UK offers plant-based detox programs to cleanse the body and energize the mind.

4. **Fitness Retreats:**

These retreats focus on physical well-being through a combination of activities such as hiking, boot camps, weight training, and cardio. They are designed to boost physical fitness, improve endurance, and promote a healthier lifestyle.

Example: BodyHoliday, located in St. Lucia, combines fitness programs with luxury spa treatments for a balanced approach to wellness.

5. **Spa and Relaxation Retreats:**

If relaxation is your main goal, spa retreats offer a range of pampering treatments, including massages, facials, and hydrotherapy. These retreats are designed to soothe the body and mind while offering a luxurious experience.

Example: Chiva-Som International Health Resort in Thailand is renowned for its spa treatments and holistic approach to relaxation and rejuvenation.

6. **Digital Detox Retreats:**

In our tech-driven world, digital detox retreats offer a break from screens and gadgets, allowing participants to reconnect with nature and themselves. These retreats often take place in remote locations where Wi-Fi and mobile phones are off-limits.

Example: Gaia Retreat & Spa in Australia encourages guests to unplug and focus on mindfulness and wellness practices.

Benefits of Attending a Wellness Retreat

Attending a wellness retreat provides transformative benefits that go beyond simple relaxation. Here are some of the key advantages:

1. **Physical Healing:**

   Retreats often include activities like yoga, hiking, or fitness training that enhance physical health. Detox and cleansing retreats help rid the body of toxins, leaving participants feeling refreshed and energized.

2. **Mental Clarity:**

   Meditation and mindfulness practices help quiet the mind and reduce stress. Participants often leave retreats with a greater sense of peace, focus, and emotional resilience.

3. **Spiritual Growth:**

   Many wellness retreats integrate spiritual practices, allowing participants to explore their inner selves and achieve personal growth. Yoga, meditation, and holistic healing can lead to deeper self-awareness and inner peace.

4. **Lifestyle Changes:**

   Retreats offer the opportunity to break old habits and create new, healthier routines. Whether it's adopting a daily meditation practice, improving your diet, or committing to regular exercise, wellness retreats help foster long-term lifestyle changes.

5. **Emotional Healing:**

   Wellness retreats provide a supportive environment for emotional healing, especially for those dealing with burnout, anxiety, or life transitions. Practices like journaling, guided therapy, or group sharing sessions offer cathartic release and self-discovery.

How to Choose the Right Wellness Retreat

With so many options available, it can be overwhelming to choose the right wellness retreat. Here are a few practical tips to help you find the perfect fit:

1. **Identify Your Goals:**

   Start by identifying what you want to achieve. Are you looking for physical fitness, mental clarity, or spiritual growth? Each retreat has its own focus, so aligning your goals with the retreat's offerings is crucial.

2. **Consider the Location:**

   Think about the type of environment that will help you relax and recharge. Do you prefer the calming sounds of the ocean, the serenity of the mountains, or the peacefulness of a forest?

3. **Review the Schedule:**

   Make sure the retreat offers activities that interest you and fit your wellness needs. Some retreats are highly structured with full-day schedules, while others offer more flexibility.

4. **Check the Expertise of Instructors:**

   The quality of the retreat largely depends on the expertise of the facilitators. Research the instructors' backgrounds to ensure they are qualified in the wellness practices being offered.

5. **Set a Budget:**

   Wellness retreats can range from budget-friendly to luxury experiences. Decide how much you're willing to spend and find a retreat that fits within your budget.

6. **Read Reviews:**

Customer reviews can provide insights into the experience offered at each retreat. Look for testimonials from past participants to get a feel for the atmosphere, quality of instruction, and overall experience.

Chapter 2:

Wellness Retreat Trends for 2025

As the wellness industry continues to grow, wellness retreats are evolving to meet the changing needs of travelers seeking rejuvenation and personal growth. 2025 is set to bring exciting new trends, as retreats around the globe embrace innovation, sustainability, and personalized wellness experiences. Whether you're looking for a digital detox, eco-friendly escape, or technology-enhanced wellness, this chapter explores the key trends shaping the world of wellness retreats in 2025.

1. Mindfulness and Mental Wellness Focus

In 2025, wellness retreats will place an even greater emphasis on mental well-being. Mindfulness practices—such as meditation, breathwork, and yoga—are becoming core elements of many retreats, offering travelers a way to disconnect from the stresses of daily life and cultivate inner peace. With increasing awareness of mental health challenges, retreats are incorporating more holistic mental wellness programs that address anxiety, depression, burnout, and emotional healing.

Example: A retreat in Sedona, Arizona, offers a 7-day mental wellness program combining mindfulness meditation, breathwork, and daily nature walks designed to improve mental clarity and emotional balance. Guests work with wellness coaches to develop practical mindfulness tools they can use long after the retreat ends.

Practical Tip:
Look for retreats that offer personalized mental health support through certified professionals, such as therapists or wellness coaches. Ask about post-retreat follow-up

services, like online mindfulness sessions, to help you integrate what you learn into your daily routine.

2. Digital Detox Escapes

With the constant bombardment of digital devices, one of the strongest trends in wellness travel for 2025 is the rise of digital detox retreats. These retreats encourage participants to completely disconnect from their phones, tablets, and laptops, allowing them to focus on the present moment. In serene natural settings, guests can restore balance by engaging in activities such as yoga, meditation, hiking, and journaling.

Example: In Costa Rica, a beachfront retreat offers a 5-day digital detox experience where guests surrender their devices upon arrival. Activities like oceanfront yoga, paddleboarding, and guided forest meditations are offered to help guests reconnect with nature and their own sense of presence.

Practical Tip:
If a full digital detox feels daunting, choose retreats that offer optional digital detox components. Start by setting specific times during your day to unplug, and gradually work toward longer periods of disconnection.

3. Sustainable and Eco-Friendly Retreats

Sustainability is no longer a trend but a necessity in the travel industry, and 2025 is seeing a surge in eco-conscious wellness retreats. These retreats prioritize environmental stewardship by using locally sourced, organic foods, renewable energy, and eco-friendly accommodations. Many are located in natural reserves or protected areas where travelers can engage in activities like forest bathing or wildlife conservation projects.

Example: A wellness retreat in Bali has implemented a zero-waste policy and features accommodations made from sustainable materials like bamboo and recycled plastics. Meals are prepared using locally grown, organic ingredients, and guests can participate in tree planting and coral reef restoration projects.

Practical Tip:

When selecting an eco-friendly retreat, research how they support sustainability. Look for certifications like LEED (Leadership in Energy and Environmental Design) or Green Globe, which guarantee environmental and social responsibility.

4. Immersive Cultural Wellness Experiences

Cultural immersion is becoming a vital aspect of wellness retreats, allowing travelers to connect deeply with the traditions, rituals, and healing practices of the destination. In 2025, more retreats are offering programs that include indigenous healing practices, spiritual ceremonies, and traditional wellness treatments such as Ayurveda, TCM (Traditional Chinese Medicine), and shamanism.

Example: A retreat in the Sacred Valley of Peru offers a transformative 10-day program that includes Andean spiritual rituals, such as coca leaf readings, sound healing with native instruments, and yoga practices combined with local healing traditions. Guests also participate in traditional temazcal (sweat lodge) ceremonies for detoxification and spiritual cleansing.

Practical Tip:

Before attending a retreat with cultural or indigenous practices, take the time to research the authenticity of the experiences offered. Choose retreats that collaborate with local communities and offer a respectful and meaningful exploration of traditional healing methods.

5. Technology-Enhanced Wellness

As technology continues to advance, some wellness retreats are incorporating it to create personalized wellness experiences. In 2025, biohacking tools, AI-powered health analysis, and virtual reality meditation are just a few ways technology is transforming retreats. These innovations help guests gain deeper insights into their health and well-being, from sleep quality and heart rate variability to stress management and dietary needs.

Example: A retreat in California offers biohacking-focused wellness programs where guests undergo a comprehensive health evaluation using AI-driven diagnostics. Based on the results, participants receive a personalized wellness plan that includes nutrition, exercise, and recovery strategies. The retreat also features high-tech amenities like cryotherapy chambers, infrared saunas, and virtual reality meditation experiences.

Practical Tip:
For those curious about technology-enhanced wellness, start by incorporating a few tech tools like wearable devices to monitor your fitness and meditation apps that guide your mindfulness practice. These tools can help you track progress both during and after your retreat.

6. Holistic Healing Through Nature

Nature-based wellness continues to be a top trend for 2025, with retreats focusing on the healing power of natural environments. From mountain retreats and forest immersions to beachfront escapes, these retreats provide an opportunity to reconnect with the Earth's rhythms, reduce stress, and boost overall well-being. Activities like forest bathing, eco-therapy, and outdoor yoga are commonly featured to help guests recharge in nature's embrace.

Example: A mountain retreat in Switzerland offers forest therapy walks where guests are guided through the serene alpine forests to connect with the natural surroundings. Daily hikes, outdoor yoga, and eco-therapy workshops are designed to reduce stress and increase a sense of well-being.

Practical Tip:

If you're planning a nature-based wellness retreat, pack light but consider bringing essentials like comfortable outdoor gear, a reusable water bottle, and a journal to document your reflections during your time in nature.

7. Personalized Wellness Journeys

In 2025, the demand for personalized wellness programs is higher than ever. Travelers are seeking retreats that offer tailored experiences based on individual goals, from stress relief and weight loss to spiritual growth and self-discovery. Wellness assessments, one-on-one consultations with experts, and customized itineraries ensure that each guest receives the specific care and attention they need.

Example: A luxury retreat in Thailand offers a bespoke wellness journey where guests work closely with nutritionists, fitness coaches, and spiritual mentors to design a fully customized retreat experience. Whether your goal is physical detox, mental clarity, or emotional healing, every aspect of your stay is tailored to help you achieve your wellness goals.

Practical Tip:

Before booking a personalized wellness retreat, make a list of your goals and desired outcomes. Discuss these with the retreat's wellness team to ensure they can provide the services and support you need for a transformative experience.

Chapter 3:

North American Wellness Retreats

North America is a diverse continent offering a range of wellness retreats designed to help you reset, recharge, and reconnect with yourself. From the vast deserts of Arizona to the serene forests of Canada, there's something for every wellness seeker. In this chapter, we'll explore some of the top wellness destinations across the USA, Canada, and Mexico, providing practical tips and examples to help you choose the perfect retreat for your needs in 2025.

1. The USA: A Wellness Haven

The United States is home to a variety of wellness retreats, each offering unique experiences, often set against breathtaking natural backdrops. Below are some of the best regions and types of retreats to consider.

California: The Land of Wellness

California is arguably the wellness capital of the United States, renowned for its progressive approach to health, fitness, and mindfulness. Retreats here cater to every type of wellness enthusiast—from yoga practitioners to detoxers.

- **Top Retreat: Esalen Institute, Big Sur** Nestled atop dramatic cliffs overlooking the Pacific Ocean, Esalen Institute is known for its holistic workshops, yoga classes, and healing hot springs. It's a transformative destination that combines personal growth with the healing power of nature.

Practical Tip: Esalen can be a splurge, but you can cut costs by booking a work-study program, where you trade volunteer hours for discounted retreat rates.

- **Top Retreat: The Ranch Malibu** This luxury boot camp retreat is ideal for those seeking a physical transformation. The Ranch offers immersive, week-long programs that include hiking, organic meals, and guided workouts, all in a stunning, secluded setting.

  Practical Tip: Book during the off-season (typically winter months) to save on rates and enjoy more personalized attention with fewer participants.

Arizona: Desert Healing

The serene desert landscape of Arizona offers an ideal environment for wellness retreats focused on spiritual healing and holistic health. Many retreats incorporate the state's Native American heritage, emphasizing spiritual renewal.

- **Top Retreat: Canyon Ranch, Tucson** Canyon Ranch is a legendary wellness resort offering personalized health programs with a focus on integrative medicine. Guests can enjoy fitness classes, nutrition consultations, and spiritual wellness activities, all set in the peaceful Arizona desert.

  Practical Tip: Canyon Ranch offers discounts for first-time visitors and special packages during shoulder seasons, like late spring and fall.

- **Top Retreat: Miraval Arizona Resort & Spa, Tucson** Known for its mindfulness and holistic wellness offerings, Miraval is perfect for those looking to disconnect and recharge. The retreat provides mindfulness activities such as guided meditation, outdoor adventure experiences, and spa treatments.

  Practical Tip: Consider visiting during one of their specialty weeks, such as "Mindfulness Month," for an enhanced focus on mental wellness.

Hawaii: Island Serenity

Hawaii's tropical climate and rich cultural heritage make it a perfect destination for those seeking relaxation and spiritual rejuvenation. Hawaiian retreats often focus on healing the body and spirit through nature immersion.

- **Top Retreat: Kalani Retreat Center, Big Island** Located on the lush, tropical Big Island, Kalani offers a mix of yoga, meditation, and cultural workshops. With an emphasis on community and nature, Kalani encourages participants to reconnect with the land and their own well-being.
  Practical Tip: Consider volunteering at Kalani for an extended stay at a reduced cost, allowing you to immerse yourself fully in the experience.

2. Canada: Nature-Focused Wellness

Canada is known for its stunning landscapes and outdoor wellness retreats, which combine nature therapy with personal development. From the forests of British Columbia to the lakes of Ontario, there are countless ways to immerse yourself in nature and find peace.

British Columbia: Forest and Ocean Retreats

British Columbia offers a unique mix of coastal retreats and forest immersion programs, where nature becomes a vital part of your wellness journey.

- **Top Retreat: Hollyhock Retreat Centre, Cortes Island** Hollyhock, located on the beautiful Cortes Island, offers a variety of wellness programs, including meditation, yoga, and personal growth workshops. The remote, oceanfront location makes it a perfect place to unplug and focus on inner well-being.
  Practical Tip: Hollyhock offers scholarships for those in need, allowing more people to experience its transformative programs at an affordable rate.

- **Top Retreat: Echo Valley Ranch & Spa, Cariboo Mountains** This luxurious yet eco-friendly ranch combines adventure with wellness, offering horseback riding, hiking, and Thai spa treatments in the heart of British Columbia's wilderness. It's ideal for those looking for a mix of nature and pampering.

  Practical Tip: Book a package deal that includes wellness services and activities to save on à la carte pricing.

Ontario: Lakeside Wellness

Ontario's serene lakes provide a tranquil setting for wellness retreats focused on mindfulness, detoxification, and outdoor activities like canoeing and hiking.

- **Top Retreat: Grail Springs Wellness Retreat, Bancroft** Grail Springs is a holistic wellness retreat set beside a crystal-clear lake, offering detox programs, meditation, and healing therapies. The focus is on physical, mental, and spiritual rejuvenation through daily activities and clean eating.

  Practical Tip: Opt for a mid-week stay to take advantage of discounted rates and avoid the busier weekend crowd.

3. Mexico: A Blend of Tradition and Modern Wellness

Mexico offers a rich blend of traditional healing methods and modern wellness approaches. Whether you're seeking a beachfront yoga retreat or a cultural healing experience, Mexico's retreats provide an opportunity to nourish both the body and the spirit.

Tulum: The Yoga Mecca

Tulum is a world-renowned destination for yoga enthusiasts, thanks to its white-sand beaches, ancient ruins, and vibrant wellness community.

- **Top Retreat: Amansala Eco-Chic Resort, Tulum** Amansala offers a unique blend of yoga, fitness, and cultural immersion. Their "Bikini Bootcamp" program combines daily workouts with yoga, while their wellness retreats focus on detoxing, relaxation, and mind-body connection.
  Practical Tip: Check the retreat calendar for special events like "Yoga Weeks" or "Detox Retreats," which often include discounted group rates.

Baja California: Luxury and Simplicity

Baja California is known for its desert-meets-ocean landscape and luxurious retreats that focus on holistic health and relaxation.

- **Top Retreat: Rancho La Puerta, Tecate** One of the world's first wellness resorts, Rancho La Puerta offers week-long retreats focusing on fitness, nutrition, and mental wellness. The program is designed to offer a complete reset for the body and mind, with activities ranging from hiking to art classes.
  Practical Tip: Rancho La Puerta offers group discounts, so consider traveling with friends or family to reduce costs.

Practical Tips for Attending North American Wellness Retreats

1. **Timing Is Key:** The best time to visit wellness retreats in North America varies by location. Desert retreats in Arizona and Mexico are best visited during the cooler months (October to April), while retreats in northern regions like Canada are more enjoyable in the summer (June to August).
2. **Budgeting:** Retreats in North America range from affordable to ultra-luxury. To save money, look for last-minute deals, off-season packages, or opt for shorter weekend retreats. Some retreats offer volunteer opportunities that allow you to participate in exchange for work.

3. **Packing Essentials:** While each retreat provides a packing list, some must-haves include comfortable clothing for yoga or fitness, reusable water bottles, eco-friendly toiletries, and a journal for reflection. Don't forget sunscreen and hiking shoes if you're attending a retreat with outdoor activities.

4. **Research Before Booking:** Before booking your retreat, read reviews and inquire about the retreat's daily schedule, meals, and accommodations to ensure it aligns with your wellness goals. Some retreats focus heavily on fitness, while others may prioritize relaxation or mental well-being.

Chapter 4:

European Escapes

Europe offers some of the most diverse and immersive wellness retreats in the world, blending rich cultural history with modern wellness practices. From the sun-soaked shores of the Mediterranean to the serene, forested landscapes of Scandinavia, Europe provides travelers with a wide range of wellness experiences tailored to body, mind, and spirit. In this chapter, we'll explore some of the best wellness retreats across Europe, offering practical tips to help you choose the perfect destination for your 2025 adventure.

1. Italy: The Heart of Wellness and Slow Living

Italy has long been synonymous with *La Dolce Vita*, or "the sweet life." It's no surprise that the country is home to a variety of wellness retreats that focus on relaxation, good food, and inner peace.

Notable Retreats:

- **Tuscany's Healing Hills:** The rolling hills of Tuscany are home to luxurious wellness retreats like **Castel Monastero**. Here, guests can enjoy personalized detox programs, yoga, and holistic therapies. The retreat also emphasizes *slow living*, where visitors disconnect from their fast-paced lives and immerse themselves in nature and local culture.
- **Amalfi Coast Spa Retreats:** For those who prefer coastal views, the Amalfi Coast is a breathtaking option. Retreats like **Monastero Santa Rosa** combine Mediterranean spa treatments with panoramic views of the sea.

Practical Tip: If you're looking for a retreat that integrates local culinary experiences, Italy's wellness retreats often feature farm-to-table meals, using organic ingredients sourced from the surrounding areas. Combine wellness with an Italian cooking class to add depth to your retreat experience.

2. Spain: The Land of Balance and Renewal

Spain is known for its vibrant culture, sunny climate, and holistic approach to wellness. Whether you're seeking mindfulness on the Mediterranean or a fitness boost in the mountains, Spain's diverse landscape offers plenty of options.

Notable Retreats:

- **Ibiza: A Mindfulness Haven:** Known for its party scene, Ibiza also has a quieter side that promotes peace and mindfulness. Wellness retreats like **Atzaró** are perfect for those looking to disconnect and rejuvenate through yoga, meditation, and spa therapies in a luxurious setting.
- **Granada: Retreats in the Sierra Nevada:** For adventure-seekers, the **Kaliyoga Retreat** in the Sierra Nevada mountains combines yoga with hiking, enabling guests to connect with nature while maintaining a focus on their wellness journey.

Practical Tip: Many Spanish retreats focus on holistic wellness, incorporating traditional Spanish practices like *siestas* (napping) and Mediterranean diets rich in olive oil, fresh vegetables, and seafood. Try to book retreats in spring or fall when the weather is ideal and fewer tourists are around.

3. Portugal: Serenity on the Atlantic

Portugal is an emerging hotspot for wellness tourism, offering retreats that emphasize mindfulness, healing, and nature. From the Algarve's sun-drenched beaches to the lush landscapes of Madeira, Portugal is a peaceful retreat destination.

Notable Retreats:

- **Algarve's Wellness by the Sea:** The southern Algarve region boasts stunning coastal retreats like **Vilalara Longevity Thalassa & Medical Spa**, where you can participate in detox programs, mindfulness workshops, and thalassotherapy (seawater therapy) sessions.
- **Madeira's Eco-Retreats:** On the island of Madeira, retreats like **Sacred Dreams Lodge** focus on eco-conscious living and wellness, offering everything from forest bathing to meditation in the island's peaceful surroundings.

Practical Tip: Portugal is known for its affordability compared to other European countries. If you're looking for a more budget-friendly wellness retreat that doesn't compromise on quality, Portugal should be on your list. Early booking, especially for retreats in the Algarve, is recommended as these spots are in high demand.

4. Greece: Ancient Healing Meets Modern Wellness

Greece has a deep history of wellness, dating back to the days of ancient healing centers like Epidaurus. Today, the country combines its ancient wisdom with modern wellness practices, offering retreats that focus on physical, emotional, and spiritual healing.

Notable Retreats:

- **Santorini's Cliffside Yoga:** Santorini is a paradise for those seeking wellness with a view. Retreats like **Andronis Concept** specialize in yoga and meditation, set against the backdrop of the island's iconic blue and white landscape.
- **Peloponnese's Spa and Nature Retreats:** In the mountainous region of the Peloponnese, retreats like **Euphoria Retreat** offer ancient Greek healing rituals combined with contemporary wellness practices, such as salt therapy and hydrotherapy.

Practical Tip: Greece is a year-round destination, but spring and autumn are the best times to visit to avoid the heat and crowds. When booking, check if the retreat offers guided tours of local historical sites—many incorporate Greek culture and history into the wellness experience, making it both enriching and healing.

5. Scandinavia: Wellness in Nature

Scandinavia's emphasis on clean living, outdoor activities, and minimalism make it a fantastic destination for wellness retreats. Whether it's forest bathing, cold-water plunges, or simply enjoying the tranquility of nature, wellness here is deeply connected to the land.

Notable Retreats:

- **Sweden's Forest Bathing and Sauna Retreats:** In Sweden, retreats like **Fjällnäs Est. 1882** offer *skogsbada* (forest bathing) and traditional Swedish saunas as part of their wellness programs. Set in remote areas, these retreats emphasize the healing power of nature and solitude.
- **Norway's Arctic Wellness:** For something truly unique, Norway's **Lyngen Lodge** offers Arctic wellness experiences, including cold-water immersion in fjords, Northern Lights meditation, and saunas in a stunning Arctic setting.

Practical Tip: Scandinavia can be expensive, but it's possible to find retreats that cater to a range of budgets. Consider visiting during the summer months for the midnight sun or winter for a chance to see the Northern Lights while practicing wellness.

6. Eastern Europe: Affordable Hidden Gems

Eastern Europe offers some of the most affordable wellness retreats in Europe, without sacrificing quality. This region is home to ancient spa towns, mineral-rich thermal waters, and traditional wellness practices that have been passed down for centuries.

Notable Retreats:

- **Hungary's Thermal Spa Towns:** Hungary's natural thermal baths are a central part of its wellness culture. Retreats in places like **Heviz Lake** offer therapeutic waters combined with yoga, detox programs, and relaxation.
- **Slovenia's Natural Wellness:** Slovenia is quickly gaining recognition for its wellness offerings. **Terme Olimia**, for example, is a luxury wellness center that features thermal baths, herbal saunas, and Ayurvedic treatments, all set in a peaceful natural environment.

Practical Tip: If you're on a budget, Eastern Europe offers great value for money. You can enjoy high-end wellness treatments at a fraction of the cost of retreats in Western Europe. Most retreats in this region include accommodation and meals, making it easier to stick to a budget.

Practical Tips for Choosing a European Wellness Retreat:

- **Timing is Key:** Europe can be crowded during the summer, so consider booking your wellness retreat in the shoulder seasons (spring or fall) for a more relaxed and intimate experience.

- **Accessibility:** Many European retreats are located in remote areas, so check transportation options before booking. Some retreats offer pick-up services from nearby airports or train stations, while others may require renting a car.

- **Cultural Experiences:** Look for retreats that incorporate local culture into their wellness programs, such as cooking classes, wine tastings, or guided historical tours. This can add a unique dimension to your retreat experience.

- **Language:** While English is widely spoken in most European countries, it's always helpful to learn a few key phrases in the local language, especially if you're venturing to more rural retreats.

Chapter 5:

Asian Serenity Retreats

Asia has long been a destination for travelers seeking spiritual awakening, holistic healing, and deep relaxation. The region's rich cultural heritage, natural beauty, and ancient wellness traditions make it an ideal place to recharge the mind, body, and soul. Whether you're looking to deepen your yoga practice in India, experience traditional healing in Thailand, or find inner peace in Japan, Asia offers a wide range of wellness retreats to suit every need. In this chapter, we will explore the best retreats across Asia, focusing on their unique offerings and practical tips to help you make the most of your wellness journey in 2025.

India: Yoga and Ayurvedic Healing

India is often considered the birthplace of wellness tourism, thanks to its centuries-old traditions of yoga and Ayurveda. For travelers seeking serenity and self-discovery, India's retreats offer a transformative experience.

Top Retreat Destinations:

- **Rishikesh:** Known as the "Yoga Capital of the World," Rishikesh, located in the foothills of the Himalayas, is home to countless yoga ashrams and meditation centers. One of the most well-known retreats is the **Ananda in the Himalayas**, which blends luxury with holistic wellness, offering yoga, Ayurveda, and meditation programs.
- **Kerala:** Kerala, located in southern India, is famous for its Ayurvedic treatments. Resorts like **Somatheeram Ayurvedic Health Resort** and **Kalari Kovilakom**

offer tailored detox programs that combine therapeutic treatments with organic food and yoga.

Practical Tips:

- **When to Go:** The best time to visit India for a wellness retreat is between November and February when the weather is cooler and pleasant.
- **What to Expect:** Daily schedules at most retreats in India typically include early morning yoga sessions, Ayurvedic consultations, meditation, and vegetarian meals.
- **Packing Essentials:** Comfortable yoga attire, sandals, and natural mosquito repellent are must-haves for retreats in India.

Thailand: Holistic and Spiritual Wellness

Thailand is known for its holistic approach to wellness, with a focus on body rejuvenation, mental clarity, and spiritual healing. Retreats here combine ancient Thai practices with modern wellness techniques, offering a unique fusion of East and West.

Top Retreat Destinations:

- **Koh Samui:** Thailand's tropical island of Koh Samui is home to world-class wellness retreats like **Kamalaya Wellness Sanctuary**. This retreat focuses on detox, stress relief, and spiritual healing, combining Thai therapies, yoga, and guided meditation.
- **Chiang Mai:** Located in northern Thailand, Chiang Mai is known for its peaceful atmosphere and lush surroundings. **The Pavana Chiang Mai Resort** offers personalized wellness programs that integrate detox, fasting, yoga, and fitness, all set against the backdrop of scenic mountain views.

Practical Tips:

- **When to Go:** The cooler months from November to February are ideal for attending a wellness retreat in Thailand, especially in the northern region.
- **Cultural Etiquette:** Thai culture emphasizes respect, particularly in spiritual and healing environments. When visiting temples or engaging in rituals, dress modestly and avoid loud or disruptive behavior.
- **Recommended Activities:** In addition to wellness programs, try a traditional Thai massage or visit a Buddhist monastery for a deeper spiritual experience.

Bali: Island Wellness and Healing

Bali, Indonesia's spiritual hub, is a go-to destination for those looking to reconnect with nature and find inner peace. The island's unique blend of natural beauty, spiritual culture, and luxury wellness offerings creates an ideal environment for personal growth and relaxation.

Top Retreat Destinations:

- **Ubud:** The cultural heart of Bali, Ubud is known for its wellness retreats, spas, and yoga centers. **The Yoga Barn** is one of the most famous retreats in Ubud, offering yoga teacher training, detox programs, and holistic healing workshops. Another popular retreat is **Fivelements Bali**, which combines ancient Balinese healing rituals with luxury spa treatments and plant-based cuisine.
- **Canggu:** A more laid-back destination, Canggu offers retreats that focus on surfing, yoga, and relaxation. **Serenity Eco Guesthouse and Yoga** is an affordable, eco-friendly retreat in Canggu that combines yoga, healthy food, and sustainable practices.

Practical Tips:

- **Best Time to Visit:** Bali's dry season from April to October is perfect for wellness retreats. During these months, you'll experience pleasant weather with minimal rainfall.
- **Health Considerations:** Bali's raw food movement is popular at wellness retreats, but if you're not used to a plant-based diet, start gradually to avoid any digestive issues.
- **Cultural Immersion:** Bali's spiritual culture is deeply ingrained in daily life. Attend a traditional Balinese purification ceremony or visit the sacred temples for a more profound cultural experience.

Japan: Zen Meditation and Onsen Relaxation

For those seeking a quieter, more introspective retreat experience, Japan offers serenity through its Zen meditation practices and hot spring (onsen) culture. Japan's retreats are perfect for those looking to disconnect from modern life and embrace simplicity and mindfulness.

Top Retreat Destinations:

- **Kyoto:** Known for its Zen gardens and Buddhist temples, Kyoto is a sanctuary for mindfulness and meditation. **The Shunkoin Temple** offers Zen meditation retreats that teach participants the art of mindfulness and inner peace through traditional Japanese practices.
- **Hakone:** Nestled near Mount Fuji, Hakone is famous for its onsens, which are natural hot springs. **Hakone Retreat Fore** is a wellness retreat that combines onsen baths with spa treatments and yoga, providing deep relaxation in a serene forest setting.

Practical Tips:

- **Etiquette:** Onsen etiquette is important in Japan. Shower and wash thoroughly before entering the communal bath, and remember to keep noise to a minimum.
- **Best Time to Go:** Spring (March to May) and autumn (September to November) offer the most pleasant weather for retreats, with beautiful cherry blossoms in spring and vibrant foliage in autumn.
- **Mindfulness Tip:** Participate in a Japanese tea ceremony during your retreat to practice mindfulness and appreciate the beauty of simplicity in everyday rituals.

Sri Lanka: Nature-Based Healing and Yoga

Sri Lanka is a rising star in the wellness world, offering retreats that focus on nature, yoga, and mindfulness. With its pristine beaches, lush jungles, and ancient healing traditions, Sri Lanka provides a perfect backdrop for transformative wellness experiences.

Top Retreat Destinations:

- **Talalla Retreat:** Situated on the southern coast of Sri Lanka, **Talalla Retreat** offers daily yoga, surf lessons, and holistic wellness programs. It's a great option for travelers looking for a blend of adventure and relaxation.
- **Sen Wellness Sanctuary:** Located in the pristine Rekawa Nature Reserve, Sen Wellness Sanctuary focuses on Ayurvedic treatments, yoga, and meditation, offering a serene setting for deep healing and self-discovery.

Practical Tips:

- **When to Visit:** The best time to visit southern Sri Lanka is from December to March, during the dry season.
- **Sustainable Travel:** Many retreats in Sri Lanka emphasize eco-conscious living. Participate in sustainability practices like beach clean-ups or support local eco-friendly businesses during your stay.

Practical Tips for Asian Serenity Retreats

1. **Research Visa Requirements:** Some Asian countries may require a visa, so be sure to check entry requirements well in advance of your trip.

2. **Book Early:** Many popular retreats in Asia fill up quickly, especially during peak seasons. Booking several months ahead can ensure you secure a spot in your preferred program.

3. **Plan for Cultural Immersion:** Take time to explore the local culture surrounding your retreat. Whether it's visiting temples, participating in local rituals, or learning traditional crafts, embracing cultural experiences will enhance your wellness journey.

4. **Health Precautions:** Make sure to check vaccination and health recommendations for each country. In tropical regions, it's important to protect against mosquito-borne illnesses like dengue or malaria.

5. **Adjust to Local Time Zones:** To combat jet lag, arrive at your destination a couple of days early and acclimate to the local time. This will allow you to start your retreat feeling refreshed and ready for mindfulness practices.

Chapter 6:

Wellness Retreats in South America

South America offers a breathtaking combination of natural beauty, ancient spirituality, and rich cultural traditions, making it a fantastic destination for wellness travelers. Whether you're looking to reconnect with nature, engage in spiritual healing, or experience unique wellness practices, this continent has something for everyone. From the Amazon rainforest's deep tranquility to the Andes Mountains' spiritual energy, South America provides an ideal setting for retreat-goers seeking rejuvenation, healing, and personal growth.

1. Why Choose South America for a Wellness Retreat?

South America's diverse landscapes and rich traditions make it one of the most captivating regions for wellness travel. The continent offers retreats in serene natural environments like rainforests, mountains, and coastlines, providing a sense of escape and rejuvenation. Moreover, many retreats are infused with ancient indigenous wisdom, offering holistic healing techniques such as shamanic rituals, traditional plant medicine, and spiritual ceremonies. For 2025, South America's wellness retreats are increasingly blending modern luxury with eco-consciousness, providing sustainable and immersive wellness experiences.

2. Top South American Wellness Retreats

a. Brazil: Nature-Focused Wellness

Brazil's vibrant culture, biodiverse landscapes, and deeply spiritual traditions make it a standout for wellness tourism. In particular, its Atlantic coastline and the Amazon rainforest provide ideal settings for healing and renewal.

- **Floripa Yoga and Surf Retreat (Florianópolis):** Situated on the idyllic island of Santa Catarina, this retreat combines daily yoga sessions with surf lessons, immersing guests in the natural beauty of Brazil's coastline. A mix of physical activity and mindfulness practices allows participants to reconnect with both body and soul, while the eco-friendly lodgings and locally sourced meals promote holistic well-being.

- **The Sanctuary in the Amazon (Manaus):** For a deeper, more spiritual experience, this retreat in the heart of the Amazon offers plant medicine ceremonies led by experienced shamans. Participants engage in Ayahuasca ceremonies, meditation, and nature walks, using the rainforest's healing energy to transform their mental, emotional, and physical well-being.

b. Peru: Spiritual Wellness in the Sacred Valley

Peru is a magnet for spiritual seekers, particularly around the Sacred Valley, which is known for its connection to ancient Incan culture. The energy of the Andes Mountains creates a powerful backdrop for healing and introspection.

- **Willka T'ika Retreat (Sacred Valley):** This luxury eco-retreat near Machu Picchu offers yoga, meditation, and chakra balancing within the Sacred Valley's mystical energy. The property features lush gardens filled with healing herbs, and guests can participate in traditional Andean ceremonies such as despacho rituals, which offer gratitude to Pachamama (Mother Earth). With its focus on spiritual and environmental harmony, Willka T'ika is ideal for those seeking both physical wellness and spiritual awakening.

- **Healing House Cusco (Cusco):** A more budget-friendly option, Healing House offers yoga, Reiki, sound healing, and workshops in the heart of Cusco. Visitors can integrate their spiritual practices with explorations of nearby Incan ruins, making for a deeply immersive experience.

c. Chile and Argentina: Luxury in the Mountains

The dramatic landscapes of Chile and Argentina provide the perfect setting for high-end wellness retreats, with their towering mountains, crystal-clear lakes, and expansive vineyards offering a sense of peaceful isolation.

- **Nayara Retreat (Patagonia, Chile):** This remote luxury retreat in Patagonia offers an extraordinary combination of wellness, adventure, and sustainability. Guests can practice yoga and mindfulness while overlooking the Andes Mountains and partake in activities like glacier hiking and horse riding. The retreat focuses on providing a digital detox, encouraging visitors to fully embrace nature and rediscover inner calm.
- **Purmamarca Retreat (Jujuy, Argentina):** Nestled in the stunning northwest region of Argentina, this wellness retreat blends modern luxury with ancient Andean traditions. Guests participate in yoga, breathwork, and mindfulness, while the nearby multicolored mountains serve as a breathtaking backdrop. Spa treatments and energy healing using local herbs and oils further enhance the experience.

d. Amazon Rainforest Retreats: Connection with Nature

For those seeking a deep connection with nature, retreats in the Amazon rainforest offer unparalleled serenity and opportunities for personal transformation. These retreats often focus on eco-conscious living, mindfulness, and healing through nature immersion.

- **Retreat Amazonia (Ecuador):** This eco-retreat offers a powerful experience centered around reconnection with nature. Guests stay in sustainably built lodges and participate in forest walks, mindfulness exercises, and yoga sessions deep within the rainforest. The retreat also provides workshops on sustainable living and local indigenous healing traditions, making it an ideal choice for environmentally conscious travelers.

3. Practical Tips for Planning a Wellness Retreat in South America

a. Best Time to Visit

South America's vast size and varied climate mean that the best time to visit depends on the location. For instance:

- **Brazil** is best visited during its dry season (April to September), particularly if you're headed to the Amazon or the coast.
- **Peru**'s Sacred Valley is ideal from May to September, as the weather is drier and sunny.
- **Chile and Argentina**'s wellness retreats are most accessible during their summer (December to February) for outdoor activities like hiking and exploring nature.

b. Budget Considerations

Wellness retreats in South America can range from affordable to high-end luxury experiences, so planning according to your budget is essential. Here's a quick overview:

- **Affordable Options:** Peru's Sacred Valley and Cusco offer budget-friendly retreats that still deliver excellent wellness experiences, with group classes and shared accommodations being more economical.
- **Luxury Options:** Chilean and Argentinean retreats tend to be more expensive, especially those in Patagonia and luxury eco-lodges in remote locations. These typically offer private accommodations, gourmet meals, and a wide range of activities.

c. Language

While many retreat centers in South America cater to international visitors and offer English-speaking staff, it's helpful to know some basic Spanish or Portuguese, especially if you're venturing into more remote areas. This will enrich your experience and make it easier to interact with locals and fully immerse yourself in the culture.

d. Health and Safety

Traveling in South America requires a few health precautions:

- **Vaccinations:** Be sure to check the recommended vaccinations for the country you're visiting. For example, **yellow fever vaccination** is often required for travel to the Amazon.
- **Travel Insurance:** Comprehensive travel insurance is a must, especially if you're engaging in outdoor activities or plant medicine ceremonies. Ensure your insurance covers any health risks that may arise during retreats.

e. Sustainability and Eco-Conscious Travel

Many wellness retreats in South America emphasize sustainability. When choosing a retreat, opt for eco-friendly options that practice responsible tourism, such as using renewable energy, offering organic meals sourced from local farms, and supporting local communities.

4. The Cultural Experience

One of the most enriching aspects of attending a wellness retreat in South America is the opportunity to engage with local traditions and cultures. Whether you participate in an **Andean despacho ceremony** in Peru or a **Candomblé ritual** in Brazil, integrating cultural elements into your wellness journey will deepen your connection to the land and its people.

Chapter 7:

Africa and Middle Eastern Wellness Retreats

The diverse landscapes, ancient healing traditions, and spiritual depth of Africa and the Middle East make this region an exceptional destination for wellness retreats. From the vast deserts of Morocco to the stunning wildlife of South Africa, and the sacred silence of Egypt's temples, these retreats offer unique experiences that blend cultural immersion, natural beauty, and rejuvenation.

In this chapter, we will explore some of the best wellness retreats in Africa and the Middle East, discuss their defining features, and offer practical tips for those looking to embark on a transformative wellness journey in this part of the world.

1. Morocco: Hammams, Yoga, and Desert Retreats

Overview: Morocco is a wellness haven, combining its ancient spa culture with modern wellness practices. The country's hammams (traditional steam baths) offer a deeply cleansing and rejuvenating experience, while the serene desert and coastal landscapes make it a perfect setting for yoga, meditation, and spiritual retreats.

Top Wellness Retreats:

- **La Pause, Marrakech Desert:** Located outside of Marrakech, La Pause offers a stunning desert retreat where guests can disconnect from the modern world and immerse themselves in the silence of the desert. The retreat focuses on mindfulness, with daily yoga sessions, guided meditation, and delicious Moroccan cuisine made from local ingredients.

- **The Kasbah Tamadot, Atlas Mountains:** Owned by Sir Richard Branson, this luxury retreat provides a combination of traditional Moroccan hammam treatments and modern spa therapies. Nestled in the High Atlas Mountains, it offers an escape into nature with its lush gardens, infinity pool, and daily yoga classes.

Practical Tips:

- **What to Expect:** Many retreats in Morocco incorporate yoga, hammam experiences, and time for reflection in breathtaking landscapes. A typical day might include a sunrise yoga session, a rejuvenating hammam, and evening meditation under the stars.
- **Travel Tip:** Marrakech is the main hub for most wellness retreats in Morocco. If you are seeking a digital detox, many desert retreats like La Pause have no Wi-Fi or electricity, which allows for complete disconnection from the outside world.

2. South Africa: Safari and Wellness Experiences

Overview: South Africa offers an unparalleled combination of adventure and wellness. Retreats here often take place in luxury safari lodges, allowing you to reconnect with nature, wildlife, and yourself. These wellness safaris combine game drives, bush walks, and outdoor yoga, providing a unique setting for personal growth and relaxation.

Top Wellness Retreats:

- **Karkloof Safari Villas, KwaZulu-Natal:** This award-winning retreat combines luxury spa treatments with the thrill of a safari. Guests can enjoy private game drives in the mornings, followed by personalized wellness therapies such as detox programs, hydrotherapy, and Ayurveda-based treatments.
- **Bushmans Kloof Wilderness Reserve, Western Cape:** Set in the stunning Cederberg Mountains, this retreat blends outdoor adventure with relaxation.

Guests can take part in ancient rock art tours, daily yoga, hiking, and indulgent spa treatments in a serene, nature-filled environment.

Practical Tips:

- **What to Expect:** Wellness safaris typically combine outdoor activities like game drives and nature walks with spa therapies and holistic healing sessions. The experience of being surrounded by wildlife in a luxurious setting makes for an unforgettable retreat.
- **Travel Tip:** South Africa's best wellness retreats are located in remote areas, so plan your travel carefully. It's a good idea to fly into Cape Town or Johannesburg and then take a domestic flight or private transfer to the retreat location.

3. Egypt: Spiritual Healing Retreats

Overview: Egypt is known for its ancient spirituality, making it a powerful destination for those seeking deep personal transformation and spiritual healing. Many wellness retreats in Egypt incorporate yoga, meditation, and mindfulness, often taking place near sacred sites like the pyramids, temples, or the Nile River.

Top Wellness Retreats:

- **Nour El Nil, Nile River Cruises:** This wellness-focused cruise along the Nile allows guests to practice yoga and meditation on the deck while floating past Egypt's most iconic historical sites. The serene setting, combined with organic meals and local cultural excursions, provides a holistic retreat experience.
- **Dahab Retreat, Sinai Peninsula:** Set on the Red Sea coast, this retreat offers a perfect blend of yoga, diving, and meditation. With the stunning backdrop of the Sinai Desert and crystal-clear waters of the Red Sea, it provides a peaceful sanctuary for those seeking both adventure and spiritual rejuvenation.

Practical Tips:

- **What to Expect:** Spiritual retreats in Egypt often focus on connecting with the country's rich history and energy. Days might include sunrise yoga, visits to temples, and guided meditations to connect with the ancient energy of the land.
- **Travel Tip:** Egypt is a popular tourist destination, so if you're seeking a more tranquil experience, look for retreats that are located outside of the major cities or offer off-peak travel times for quieter settings.

4. Wellness in the Arabian Desert

Overview: The Arabian Desert offers a unique wellness experience, with its vast, untouched landscapes providing a sense of peace and tranquility. Many wellness retreats in the Middle East, particularly in the UAE and Oman, focus on luxury, offering world-class spa services, yoga, and meditation sessions against the backdrop of sand dunes and starry skies.

Top Wellness Retreats:

- **Al Maha Desert Resort, UAE:** Located in the Dubai Desert Conservation Reserve, Al Maha offers a luxury wellness experience like no other. With desert views, camel treks, and private spa services, this resort allows guests to experience the serenity of the desert while indulging in high-end wellness treatments.
- **Six Senses Zighy Bay, Oman:** Nestled between the mountains and the sea, this luxury retreat offers a combination of desert and coastal wellness experiences. Daily yoga, meditation, and detox programs are complemented by a variety of outdoor activities like paragliding and snorkeling.

Practical Tips:

- **What to Expect:** Retreats in the Arabian Desert focus on indulgence, with luxury spas, personalized wellness programs, and outdoor activities that encourage connection with nature. The desert's stillness makes it an ideal place for deep relaxation and inner reflection.
- **Travel Tip:** Most desert retreats in the UAE and Oman are located near major cities like Dubai and Muscat. Make sure to book in advance, as these retreats are popular during the cooler months (October to March).

Practical Tips for Wellness Retreats in Africa and the Middle East

1. **Best Time to Visit:**
   - Africa and the Middle East can be extremely hot during the summer months (June to August). The best time to visit for wellness retreats is generally from October to March, when temperatures are more comfortable.
2. **What to Pack:**
   - Lightweight, breathable clothing is essential, especially for desert retreats. Don't forget sunscreen, a wide-brimmed hat, and comfortable yoga wear. For safaris, pack neutral-colored clothing to blend in with the environment.
3. **Cultural Sensitivity:**
   - Both Africa and the Middle East have rich cultural traditions. When attending retreats, be mindful of local customs, especially in the Middle East, where modest dress and conservative behavior may be required in public spaces.
4. **Traveling Safely:**
   - Ensure you have the necessary vaccinations for certain parts of Africa. In more remote areas, it's a good idea to bring a basic first aid kit and any personal medications. Check travel advisories before booking your trip.

Chapter 8:

Oceania's Wellness Havens

Oceania, with its pristine landscapes and laid-back lifestyle, is a haven for those seeking a rejuvenating escape. From the lush rainforests and dramatic coastlines of New Zealand to Australia's golden beaches and the tranquil islands of the South Pacific, this region offers diverse wellness experiences. Whether you're seeking adventure, relaxation, or spiritual renewal, Oceania has something to suit every wellness traveler.

Why Oceania?

Oceania's wellness retreats are defined by their deep connection to nature, an emphasis on outdoor activities, and a focus on sustainable living. The region's indigenous cultures also play a role, infusing ancient practices into modern wellness experiences. With the growing trend of eco-friendly retreats and a strong focus on sustainability, Oceania stands out as a perfect destination for wellness seekers in 2025.

1. Australia: Beachfront Wellness and Eco-Retreats

Australia is a prime destination for wellness retreats, offering a wide array of experiences, from luxury beachfront resorts to immersive eco-friendly escapes. Wellness tourism here centers around nature, mindfulness, and a sense of adventure.

Popular Destinations:

- **Byron Bay, New South Wales**

  Known as Australia's wellness capital, Byron Bay is a must-visit for those looking to unwind in a relaxed, bohemian setting. You'll find a variety of retreats here offering yoga, meditation, and detox programs. One of the top choices is **Gaia Retreat & Spa**, co-founded by Olivia Newton-John, which offers personalized wellness programs including yoga, meditation, and organic meals sourced from their on-site garden.

  Practical Tip: Byron Bay is busiest during the summer months (December to February), so consider visiting during the shoulder seasons (March-May, September-November) for a more peaceful experience.

- **Great Barrier Reef, Queensland**

  Combine wellness with underwater adventures at retreats along the Great Barrier Reef. Luxury resorts such as **Qualia on Hamilton Island** blend relaxation with marine exploration, offering yoga classes, spa treatments, and guided snorkeling or diving tours. The retreat's serene surroundings make it an ideal spot for mental and physical rejuvenation.

  Practical Tip: Book snorkeling or diving tours in advance to ensure availability, especially during peak travel seasons (June to October).

- **Tasmania**

  For a more nature-immersive experience, Tasmania's untouched wilderness is home to eco-friendly wellness retreats that emphasize sustainability. **Saffire Freycinet** offers holistic wellness experiences, combining spa treatments, mindful nature walks, and locally sourced organic cuisine. Visitors can hike through Freycinet National Park, known for its breathtaking views, while focusing on mindfulness and grounding practices.

  Practical Tip: Pack layered clothing when visiting Tasmania, as the weather can change rapidly, even in summer.

2. New Zealand: Adventure and Wellness in Nature

New Zealand, renowned for its natural beauty, offers wellness retreats that integrate adventure and relaxation. From the geothermal hot springs of Rotorua to the stunning fjords of the South Island, New Zealand is perfect for those who want to combine outdoor activities with wellness practices.

Popular Destinations:

- **Queenstown, South Island**

  Queenstown is known as the adventure capital of New Zealand, and its wellness retreats reflect this, combining thrilling outdoor activities with relaxation. **Aro Hā Wellness Retreat** is one of the top-rated retreats in the region, offering yoga, meditation, and wellness programs alongside hiking, kayaking, and other outdoor adventures. The retreat is designed for those seeking a transformative experience, blending physical challenge with mindfulness.

  Practical Tip: Due to its popularity, Aro Hā books up quickly, so plan and reserve your spot at least 6 months in advance, especially for the high season (December to March).

- **Rotorua, North Island**

  Famed for its geothermal activity, Rotorua is a wellness hub in New Zealand. The **Polynesian Spa** is a well-known retreat that uses the natural geothermal waters for healing and relaxation. Guests can soak in the therapeutic hot pools while enjoying lake views, and choose from a variety of wellness treatments, including mud baths and mineral-infused therapies.

  Practical Tip: Allow time to explore the nearby geothermal parks and cultural sites, which provide insight into Māori traditions and their connection to wellness.

3. Fiji and the South Pacific Islands: Island Wellness Escapes

The South Pacific islands, including Fiji, Tahiti, and the Cook Islands, are famous for their pristine beaches, crystal-clear waters, and relaxed island atmosphere. Wellness retreats in this region focus on the healing power of the ocean, indigenous healing practices, and luxury relaxation.

Popular Destinations:

- **Fiji**

  Fiji's luxury wellness retreats are designed to nourish both body and mind, with most retreats offering beachfront yoga, spa treatments, and wellness activities focused on natural healing. **Koro Sun Resort & Rainforest Spa** on Vanua Levu is a standout retreat, offering holistic programs that blend Fijian traditions with modern wellness practices. The resort's signature treatments incorporate local ingredients like coconut and sugar cane to rejuvenate the skin and body.

  Practical Tip: Consider staying at an all-inclusive resort to ensure that meals, activities, and treatments are included, making budgeting easier.

- **Tahiti, French Polynesia**

  Tahiti and its neighboring islands are often seen as paradise on earth. Wellness retreats like **The Brando** offer eco-friendly luxury in an intimate island setting. This resort emphasizes sustainability and features spa treatments inspired by Polynesian traditions, including the use of local vanilla and coconut oils for massage.

  Practical Tip: For a quieter experience, visit during the low season (November to March), but be aware of increased rain during this period.

- **Cook Islands**

  For a more off-the-beaten-path wellness escape, the Cook Islands provide serenity and natural beauty without the large tourist crowds. **Aitutaki Lagoon Private Island Resort** offers an ideal mix of beachside yoga, snorkeling, and traditional

Polynesian spa treatments. The peaceful environment allows for a deeper connection to nature and self.

Practical Tip: Island-hopping is popular in the Cook Islands, so plan excursions to explore different parts of this tropical paradise during your stay.

Practical Tips for Wellness Travelers in Oceania

- **Seasonal Considerations:** The peak travel season in Oceania is during the summer months (December to February), so if you prefer quieter retreats and lower costs, consider traveling during the shoulder seasons (March-May, September-November). Be mindful of weather patterns, especially in tropical areas where rainy seasons can affect travel.

- **Travel Logistics:** Oceania is a large region, and traveling between islands or countries can be time-consuming. Plan your itinerary carefully to minimize travel fatigue. Domestic flights in Australia and New Zealand are common, and many South Pacific islands have small airports served by regional airlines.

- **Sustainability:** Many retreats in Oceania emphasize eco-friendliness and sustainability. Opt for retreats that prioritize environmental responsibility, from energy use to locally sourced organic food. Not only will this enhance your wellness experience, but it will also reduce your travel footprint.

- **Packing Essentials:** Given the diverse climates, pack lightweight, breathable clothing for warmer coastal areas, and layered outfits for cooler regions like New Zealand's South Island or Tasmania. Don't forget sunscreen, insect repellent, and sturdy shoes for nature-based activities.

Chapter 9:

What to Expect at a Wellness Retreat

Whether you're embarking on your first wellness retreat or you're a seasoned traveler, understanding what awaits you is essential for maximizing the benefits of your experience. Wellness retreats vary greatly in their offerings, atmosphere, and goals, but most share common elements designed to nurture your mind, body, and spirit. In this chapter, we'll explore what a typical day at a retreat looks like, what activities and amenities you might find, and how to mentally and physically prepare yourself for the experience.

1. A Typical Day at a Wellness Retreat

Most wellness retreats offer structured daily schedules that blend relaxation, personal development, and physical activity. While the exact program will depend on the theme of the retreat (e.g., yoga, meditation, detox), there are some general patterns you can expect:

- **Morning: Mindful Start**
  - Most wellness retreats kick off the day with some form of mindfulness practice, such as meditation or yoga. For example, retreats in Bali or Thailand might begin with sunrise yoga sessions overlooking tranquil beaches or rice fields. The focus is on centering the mind and body, setting a peaceful tone for the day.
  - **Tip:** Arrive at the morning session early, as this is often the time when you'll feel most connected to the surroundings and fellow participants. Dress comfortably and consider bringing your own yoga mat for extra comfort.

- **Mid-Morning: Nourishing Breakfast**
  - Following your morning practice, expect a nutritious and often plant-based breakfast. Meals are typically designed to support wellness goals, focusing on fresh, organic ingredients. Retreats in places like California and Spain often emphasize farm-to-table dining, with locally sourced ingredients prepared by gourmet chefs.
  - **Tip:** If you have dietary restrictions or preferences, notify the retreat ahead of time. Many retreats are happy to accommodate vegetarian, vegan, gluten-free, or other specialized diets.
- **Midday: Workshops, Excursions, or Healing Sessions**
  - After breakfast, most retreats schedule personal development workshops, fitness classes, or excursions. For example, a detox retreat might include a guided nature hike followed by a juicing workshop, while a meditation retreat could offer mindfulness classes and group discussions on mental clarity.
  - Depending on the location, you might also engage in cultural or environmental activities, like visiting nearby landmarks or participating in community service. Retreats in Peru or India might take participants on excursions to sacred sites, blending wellness with cultural immersion.
  - **Tip:** If the retreat offers multiple sessions or activities, try to balance between physically demanding and more restful sessions. Overextending yourself may reduce your ability to fully relax and absorb the experience.
- **Afternoon: Leisure or Spa Treatments**
  - The afternoons are typically more relaxed, offering personal time for spa treatments, journaling, or solo reflection. Many retreats boast world-class spas, offering massages, facials, body scrubs, and more. For instance, luxury retreats in Morocco or the Maldives often include Hammam experiences, where the body is scrubbed and cleansed in a traditional steam bath.

- ○ **Tip:** Book spa treatments early, as these sessions tend to fill up quickly. Consider scheduling them toward the end of your stay to further enhance the relaxation process after you've settled into the retreat.
- **Evening: Group Dinners and Evening Practice**
  - ○ Dinners at wellness retreats are usually communal, offering a chance to bond with fellow participants over wholesome meals. It's an opportunity to reflect on the day's experiences and share insights. After dinner, some retreats will have a gentle evening yoga session, meditation, or sound healing, such as Tibetan bowl therapy.
  - ○ **Tip:** Don't feel pressured to be overly social during meal times if you need quiet reflection. Most retreat environments are respectful of personal boundaries, so it's okay to excuse yourself or sit quietly.

2. Accommodations and Amenities

The type of accommodation will depend on the retreat's location and theme. From luxury villas in Bali to eco-lodges in Costa Rica, wellness retreats offer a range of options to suit various tastes and budgets. Here's a breakdown of what you might expect:

- **Private vs. Shared Rooms**
  - ○ Many retreats offer both private and shared accommodations. Private rooms are ideal if you're seeking solitude and personal reflection, while shared rooms provide a sense of community and can be more budget-friendly.
  - ○ **Tip:** If you're sharing a room, pack lightly and be considerate of your roommate's personal space. Noise-cancelling headphones and an eye mask can help ensure restful sleep.
- **On-site Spa and Wellness Facilities**

- High-end wellness retreats often boast luxurious spa facilities, with pools, saunas, steam rooms, and fitness centers. You may also find holistic treatments like acupuncture, Reiki, or energy healing.
  - **Tip:** Take advantage of free amenities such as saunas and steam rooms, which can enhance relaxation and detoxification during your stay.
- **Connection to Nature**
  - Many wellness retreats are set in serene, nature-rich environments. Whether it's a beachfront property in Hawaii, a mountain lodge in the Alps, or a jungle hideaway in Costa Rica, expect to spend significant time outdoors. Activities often include hiking, nature walks, or even meditative beach sessions.
  - **Tip:** Bring appropriate gear for outdoor activities, such as hiking shoes, swimsuits, or insect repellent, depending on the environment.

3. Food and Nutrition: Fueling Your Wellness Journey

The food served at wellness retreats plays a pivotal role in the experience. You can expect meals designed to nourish and detoxify your body, often using organic, local, and seasonal ingredients.

- **Detox Diets and Cleanses**
  - Many retreats offer specialized detox diets or cleanses, which could involve plant-based meals, juices, or even fasting periods. Retreats in Thailand or Costa Rica are known for their detox programs, which aim to eliminate toxins and reset the body.
  - **Tip:** If you're participating in a detox or cleanse, stay hydrated and listen to your body. Sudden changes in diet may initially cause discomfort, but the retreat will often provide supportive guidance.

- **Gourmet Wellness**
  - On the other end of the spectrum, some retreats, especially those in Europe or California, take pride in offering gourmet wellness cuisine. Here, you'll enjoy balanced meals that are both nutritious and indulgent, often prepared by chefs with a focus on superfoods and gut health.
  - **Tip:** Embrace trying new flavors and ingredients that you may not be accustomed to. Retreats often introduce participants to healthier alternatives to everyday foods.

4. Preparing for Your Retreat

Being mentally and physically prepared for your wellness retreat can help you fully embrace the experience. Here are some key tips:

- **Packing Essentials**
  - Aside from comfortable clothing, consider packing a journal for reflection, reusable water bottles, comfortable shoes for walking or hiking, and personal wellness items like essential oils or a travel yoga mat.
  - **Tip:** Don't overpack. Many retreats encourage minimalism to help participants disconnect from material clutter.
- **Mindset and Intentions**
  - Approach your retreat with clear intentions. Whether you're there to relax, heal, or grow, having a focused mindset will help you gain the most from the experience. You might want to journal before the retreat, noting personal goals or areas you'd like to work on during your stay.
  - **Tip:** Allow yourself to be open to new experiences, even if they feel out of your comfort zone. Wellness retreats are designed to gently push you toward personal growth.

5. Unplugging and Digital Detox

A key element of many wellness retreats is disconnecting from the digital world. Many retreats, especially those focused on mindfulness, encourage a full digital detox, which means leaving your phone, laptop, and other devices behind.

- **Tip:** If going entirely offline feels daunting, consider a gradual detox by limiting your device usage to a specific time of day. Inform family and friends ahead of time so they understand that you'll be largely unreachable.

Chapter 10:

Budgeting for Your Wellness Retreat

Planning a wellness retreat can be an incredibly rewarding experience, but it's essential to ensure that the costs align with your budget. While the idea of escaping to a peaceful destination to recharge your mind, body, and soul is appealing, the financial aspect can sometimes feel overwhelming. Fortunately, there are ways to manage your spending without sacrificing the quality of your experience. This chapter will guide you through the essentials of budgeting for your wellness retreat in 2025, offering practical tips and examples to help you stay on track.

1. Understanding the Costs of a Wellness Retreat

Wellness retreats come in a variety of price ranges, from budget-friendly getaways to high-end luxury experiences. Before you start planning, it's important to understand what you're paying for. Here's a breakdown of the typical expenses associated with a retreat:

- **Accommodation**: This is often the largest portion of the retreat's cost. Luxury resorts with spa services and organic dining will charge more than rustic retreats or community-driven wellness centers.
- **Meals**: Most wellness retreats include meals in the package, but the type of cuisine and dietary options can affect the cost. Gourmet, organic, and detox-specific meals are typically more expensive.
- **Workshops and Activities**: Yoga classes, meditation sessions, wellness workshops, and other activities may be included in the price or offered as optional add-ons. Retreats offering specialized or exclusive experiences (e.g., sound healing, private fitness coaching) tend to be pricier.

- **Transportation**: Flights, airport transfers, and ground transportation can vary significantly depending on the destination.
- **Extras and Amenities**: Massages, spa treatments, and excursions are often offered as optional services, and these can quickly add up if not planned for.

2. Setting a Realistic Budget

When budgeting for your wellness retreat, it's crucial to set a realistic financial limit that works for you. Here's a step-by-step guide to help you plan:

- **Determine Your Overall Spending Limit**: Start by identifying the total amount you're willing to spend, including all aspects of the retreat. Be honest with yourself about your financial situation and ensure this amount won't strain other areas of your life.
- **Break Down Your Costs**: Divide your budget into categories—accommodation, travel, meals, activities, and extras. Having a clear understanding of where your money will go helps avoid surprises later on.
  Example:
  If your total budget is $3,000, you might allocate $1,500 for accommodation, $500 for meals, $700 for travel, and $300 for extras like spa treatments or excursions.
- **Build in a Buffer**: Unexpected expenses are common during travel, so add a 10–15% buffer to your budget to cover any unforeseen costs.

3. Choosing Between Affordable and Luxury Retreats

The wellness retreat industry caters to a wide range of budgets, so it's important to choose an option that aligns with your financial capabilities.

- **Budget-Friendly Retreats**: These typically include group accommodations, simpler meals, and basic wellness activities such as yoga and meditation. They often take place in local or rural settings, such as farm stays or nature camps, which can help reduce costs. You'll likely be sharing spaces with other attendees, which fosters a sense of community while cutting down expenses.

  Example:

  A 7-day yoga retreat in Costa Rica at an eco-lodge might cost around $1,000–$1,500, including shared accommodation, vegetarian meals, and daily yoga classes.

- **Luxury Wellness Retreats**: For those willing to splurge, high-end retreats offer private villas, gourmet organic meals, spa services, and personalized wellness programs. The locations are often exclusive, such as private islands or resorts in scenic, exotic locales. While the experience is undoubtedly lavish, these retreats can cost anywhere from $5,000 to $10,000 or more.

  Example:

  A luxury retreat in Bali might feature private villas, a personal wellness concierge, daily spa treatments, and premium organic meals, priced at $7,000 for a 10-day stay.

4. Hidden Costs to Watch For

Even after you've booked your retreat, there are often hidden costs that can catch you off guard. Here are a few to keep in mind:

- **Airport Transfers**: Some retreats offer free shuttle services, but many require you to arrange your own transportation. If your retreat is in a remote location, taxi or private transfer costs can add up.

Tip: Always check if airport transfers are included in the package. If not, consider ride-sharing apps or public transport to save money.

- **Taxes and Resort Fees**: Certain retreats may not include taxes, service charges, or resort fees in the listed price. These can add an extra 10-20% to your total bill.
  Tip: Always read the fine print and factor in taxes and fees when budgeting.

- **Gratuities**: Many retreats do not include gratuities for staff in their prices, and tipping can be a significant extra cost. Spa staff, housekeeping, and restaurant workers typically expect gratuities, especially in luxury settings.
  Tip: Research the local tipping customs ahead of time and set aside a portion of your budget for this.

5. Finding Deals and Discounts

There are several ways to save money on a wellness retreat, even if you're looking at higher-end destinations.

- **Off-Peak Travel**: Prices for wellness retreats can fluctuate dramatically depending on the season. Traveling during the off-peak season (when fewer tourists visit) can save you a significant amount on accommodation and travel.
  Example:
  A retreat in Bali might be $3,000 during the high season (June-August), but in the rainy season (October-March), the price could drop to $2,000 or less.

- **Last-Minute Deals**: Some retreat centers offer last-minute discounts if they have open spots. This can be a great way to attend a high-quality retreat for a lower price.
  Tip: Sign up for newsletters or follow retreat centers on social media to stay informed about special promotions or last-minute openings.

- **Early-Bird Discounts**: Many retreats offer early booking discounts if you reserve your spot several months in advance. This is a smart way to lock in a lower price. **Tip**: If you know your travel dates and destination in advance, take advantage of early-bird offers, which can save you anywhere from 10-30%.

6. Tips for Budgeting Your Travel Costs

Traveling to your retreat can represent a significant portion of your budget, especially if the destination is remote or international. Here are some practical tips for keeping travel costs down:

- **Book Flights Early**: Airfare tends to rise as the departure date approaches, so book your flights as early as possible to get the best rates.
- **Use Travel Points or Rewards**: If you have a credit card with travel rewards, consider using points to cover flights, hotels, or even retreat costs.
- **Look for Alternative Airports**: Flying into a nearby, less popular airport can sometimes save hundreds of dollars.
  Example:
  If your retreat is in the south of France, consider flying into a nearby country like Spain or Italy and taking a train, which could save money on airfare.

7. Maximizing Your Retreat Experience on a Budget

Even if you're attending a more affordable retreat, there are ways to maximize your experience without overspending:

- **Focus on Free Activities**: Take full advantage of any included wellness activities, such as guided nature walks, group meditations, or yoga classes, instead of paying for extra workshops or spa treatments.
- **Stay Longer for Less**: Some retreats offer reduced daily rates if you stay for an extended period (e.g., 10 days instead of 5). If your schedule allows, this could be a great way to get more value for your money.

Chapter 11:

Making the Most of Your Retreat

Attending a wellness retreat is a transformative experience, but making the most out of it requires more than just showing up. It's about embracing the opportunity for growth, healing, and self-discovery. In this chapter, we'll explore practical tips and strategies to maximize the benefits of your retreat, ensuring you return home rejuvenated, recharged, and ready to continue your wellness journey.

1. Set Clear Intentions Before You Arrive

Before stepping foot on your retreat, take time to reflect on what you hope to achieve. Are you looking to reduce stress, reconnect with nature, improve your physical health, or deepen your meditation practice? Setting clear intentions will guide your experience, helping you focus on the areas of your life you wish to nurture.

- **Tip:** Write down 2-3 personal goals. For example, "I want to learn how to meditate daily" or "I want to disconnect from technology and be present in the moment."
- **Example:** Samantha attended a week-long yoga retreat in Costa Rica with the intention of overcoming burnout. By clearly defining her goal to unwind and practice mindfulness, she was able to focus on yoga and breathing exercises that helped her find inner peace.

2. Embrace the Retreat Schedule, but Be Flexible

Wellness retreats often have structured daily schedules, including morning meditations, afternoon workshops, and evening discussions. While it's important to participate in these activities to fully immerse yourself, give yourself permission to take breaks if needed. Listen to your body and mind—sometimes resting is as essential as engaging.

- **Tip:** If the retreat offers free time or optional activities, use this time to reflect, journal, or simply rest. Don't feel pressured to attend every session if you're feeling overwhelmed.
- **Example:** During a retreat in the mountains of Colorado, Ben felt exhausted after several intense hiking sessions. Instead of forcing himself to join a meditation class, he opted for a quiet walk through the forest, which gave him the solitude and reflection he needed.

3. Participate Fully in Activities and Workshops

One of the greatest benefits of a wellness retreat is the opportunity to try new things. Whether it's a group yoga session, a sound healing workshop, or an Ayurvedic cooking class, participating fully in these activities opens the door to new experiences that could become part of your daily routine once you return home.

- **Tip:** Approach every activity with an open mind, even if it feels unfamiliar or outside of your comfort zone. This is where growth happens.
- **Example:** At a meditation retreat in Thailand, Julie initially struggled with sitting in silence for long periods. However, after attending a guided walking meditation class, she discovered a new practice that she enjoyed and incorporated into her life after the retreat.

4. Disconnect from Technology and Reconnect with Yourself

Most wellness retreats encourage guests to limit or entirely disconnect from technology to help them focus on their surroundings and inner self. Embrace this opportunity to unplug from daily distractions. This break from emails, social media, and constant notifications is essential to fully engage in the retreat's offerings.

- **Tip:** Turn off your phone or keep it in airplane mode for the duration of the retreat, only using it when absolutely necessary. Instead, journal your thoughts, read, or simply observe the beauty around you.
- **Example:** Jacob attended a digital detox retreat in Bali where participants handed over their devices upon arrival. Without his phone, he found himself more attuned to the sounds of nature, the taste of meals, and the depth of conversations with fellow attendees.

5. Cultivate Mindfulness and Presence

Wellness retreats are the perfect environment to practice mindfulness—being fully present in each moment. Whether you're meditating, walking, eating, or interacting with others, focus on your breath, your surroundings, and your sensations.

- **Tip:** During meals, practice mindful eating by paying attention to each bite, savoring the flavors and textures. This simple practice can enhance your relationship with food and make meals more enjoyable and fulfilling.
- **Example:** At a retreat in the French countryside, Rachel learned mindful eating techniques that helped her reduce stress around food. By slowing down and appreciating every bite, she found joy in her meals, a practice she continued long after returning home.

6. Connect with Fellow Attendees

Retreats attract people who are also on their wellness journey, and connecting with others can add immense value to your experience. Sharing stories, supporting each other's goals, and learning from different perspectives can create lasting friendships and enrich your stay.

- **Tip:** Engage in group activities and meals where conversations flow naturally. Share your experiences and be open to learning from others. Some of the best lessons come from fellow retreat-goers.
- **Example:** During a mindfulness retreat in Sedona, Arizona, David formed a close bond with a fellow participant who introduced him to new breathing techniques. Their friendship continued post-retreat, and they now practice together virtually.

7. Be Open to Emotional and Physical Breakthroughs

Wellness retreats can evoke powerful emotional and physical changes. As you engage in deep reflection, meditation, or healing therapies, it's normal to experience a range of emotions—from joy to vulnerability. Allow yourself to feel and process these emotions, as they are a natural part of growth.

- **Tip:** If you experience an emotional release during the retreat, don't suppress it. Speak to facilitators or guides who can offer support and insight. Journaling is also an excellent way to process emotions.
- **Example:** During a retreat in Peru, Vanessa experienced a deep emotional release while participating in a cacao ceremony. Though unexpected, she felt lighter and more connected to herself after allowing those emotions to surface and be expressed.

8. Reflect and Journal Your Experience

Documenting your thoughts, emotions, and experiences throughout the retreat can help you internalize the lessons you're learning. Journaling provides a safe space for reflection and can serve as a valuable tool when you return home, allowing you to revisit your retreat journey whenever needed.

- **Tip:** Set aside 10-15 minutes each day to journal. Write about how you're feeling, the activities you've participated in, and any breakthroughs or challenges you've faced.
- **Example:** Claire found that keeping a journal during her silent retreat in the Swiss Alps allowed her to process the silence and isolation more deeply. After the retreat, reading her entries helped her continue the mindfulness practices she learned.

9. Integrate Wellness Practices into Daily Life After the Retreat

The true success of a wellness retreat lies in how you integrate its teachings into your everyday life. To maintain the momentum, create a plan for incorporating what you've learned—whether it's a new meditation routine, healthier eating habits, or regular yoga practice.

- **Tip:** Set small, realistic goals for yourself post-retreat, like meditating for 10 minutes each morning or eating mindfully during one meal a day. Gradually, these small practices will become a natural part of your routine.
- **Example:** After a week-long yoga retreat in Hawaii, Melissa set a goal to practice yoga for 20 minutes every morning. By starting small, she was able to maintain a consistent practice and noticed the benefits in both her physical and mental well-being.

Chapter 12:

Bonus Tips for Wellness Travelers

Wellness travel is more than just a vacation—it's a transformative journey toward greater health, mindfulness, and personal growth. Whether you're a seasoned wellness traveler or embarking on your first retreat, there are several ways to enhance your experience and make the most of your time away. In this chapter, we'll share some bonus tips for wellness travelers that will help you prepare mentally, physically, and emotionally for your next adventure.

1. Solo Travel vs. Group Retreats: Pros and Cons

Solo Travel

Traveling solo for a wellness retreat can be an empowering experience. It allows you to focus entirely on your personal growth without the distractions of companions. Many people choose to travel solo when they are seeking time for self-reflection, healing, or personal discovery.

Pros:

- Complete flexibility in choosing your retreat and schedule.
- Opportunities for deep personal reflection and growth.
- Easier to meet new people and engage with others at the retreat.

  Cons:

- Loneliness may be a challenge if you prefer social interaction.
- Higher cost, as you won't have anyone to share accommodation or transportation expenses.
- No travel companion to assist in unfamiliar environments.

Example:

Sarah, a busy professional, felt overwhelmed by her work life and decided to take a solo trip to a yoga retreat in Bali. Without the obligations of traveling with friends or family, she could completely immerse herself in the healing practices offered. She returned home feeling more centered and capable of balancing her career with self-care.

Group Travel

Group retreats can offer a sense of camaraderie and shared experience, which can be deeply fulfilling. Many retreats cater to specific groups such as couples, friends, or even strangers who bond over shared goals like fitness or meditation.

Pros:

- Built-in social interaction and support from fellow travelers.
- Group activities can enhance the experience through shared learning.
- Lower costs for accommodations and group activities.

Cons:

- Less personal time and flexibility to follow your own schedule.
- Group dynamics may not always suit your personal energy.
- May feel restricted if you're an introvert or prefer more solitude.

Example:

A group of friends from New York decided to attend a wellness retreat in Sedona, Arizona. They enjoyed the group activities, such as guided hikes and meditations, and felt that the experience brought them closer as friends. Additionally, the shared cost of accommodations made it more affordable for everyone.

2. How to Stay Safe and Healthy While Traveling

Traveling for a wellness retreat can sometimes come with its own set of challenges, especially when you're navigating unfamiliar locations. Keeping yourself safe and healthy should always be a top priority.

Health Tips:

- **Hydration:** Many retreats are in hot or tropical climates, making hydration essential. Carry a refillable water bottle, especially during outdoor activities like hiking or yoga.
- **Vaccinations and Medications:** Depending on where you're traveling, check for required vaccinations. Also, pack any necessary medications and basic first-aid supplies like bandages, pain relievers, and hand sanitizer.
- **Insurance:** Ensure you have appropriate travel insurance that covers medical emergencies, especially if you're attending retreats in remote areas.

Safety Tips:

- **Research your destination:** Before you travel, research the area to understand any local risks, from weather conditions to cultural norms.
- **Secure your belongings:** Keep your travel documents, money, and other valuables in a secure place, such as a money belt or a locked bag in your accommodation.
- **Know local emergency contacts:** Familiarize yourself with local emergency numbers and the location of nearby medical facilities.
- **Stay connected:** Let someone back home know your itinerary and check in regularly.

3. Best Times of the Year to Travel for Wellness

The timing of your wellness retreat can greatly affect your experience, especially in terms of weather, costs, and availability.

- **Peak Season:** During the peak season (e.g., summer and holiday periods), wellness retreats can be more expensive and crowded. However, this is also when retreats offer a full range of activities and workshops, so it can be ideal if you're looking for a vibrant and energetic environment.
- **Off-Peak Season:** Traveling during the off-peak season can lead to significant savings. Many retreats offer discounts during these periods, and the atmosphere tends to be more relaxed and less crowded. However, some activities may be limited due to weather or staff availability.

Example:

For a yoga retreat in Costa Rica, the dry season (December to April) is considered the peak season with sunny weather, but it's also the most expensive time to visit. Opting for the rainy season (May to November) may mean occasional showers, but you'll enjoy lush green landscapes, lower prices, and fewer crowds.

4. Insider Tips for an Enhanced Retreat Experience

Set Personal Goals and Intentions

Before arriving at your wellness retreat, take some time to set clear personal goals and intentions. Whether it's stress reduction, physical healing, spiritual growth, or simply disconnecting from everyday life, having clear objectives will help you get the most out of your experience. Write down your goals in a journal and revisit them throughout your stay.

Engage Fully in the Experience

Embrace the retreat's offerings with an open mind and heart. Participate in activities even if they are new or challenging. Whether it's a silent meditation, an unfamiliar fitness class, or a new dietary regime, these experiences are designed to push you out of your comfort zone and foster growth. Be present and open to the lessons that arise.

Example:

At a mindfulness retreat in India, participants were encouraged to practice noble silence—remaining silent for several days to cultivate inner peace. At first, many found it difficult, but by the end of the retreat, they experienced profound clarity and emotional healing through the practice.

Disconnect from Technology

Wellness retreats are the perfect opportunity to unplug from the constant distractions of modern life. Many retreats encourage guests to limit their use of phones, laptops, and other devices. By disconnecting, you'll create space for introspection, relaxation, and meaningful connections with others.

Integrating Wellness Practices Post-Retreat

One of the challenges after returning home is maintaining the positive habits and mindset cultivated during the retreat. Make a plan to integrate key practices into your daily routine, whether it's a morning meditation, regular yoga sessions, or mindful eating habits. Use reminders, apps, or even accountability partners to stay on track.

Example:

After a week-long detox retreat in California, John committed to continuing his daily meditation practice. He set a 10-minute timer every morning to meditate before starting his day, which helped him stay grounded and focused even months after the retreat.

5. Packing Essentials for Wellness Retreats

Packing wisely can make a big difference in your comfort and overall experience at a wellness retreat. Here are some essentials to consider:

- **Clothing:** Opt for lightweight, breathable clothing suitable for yoga, hiking, or meditation sessions. Pack layers if you're attending a retreat in a place with varying temperatures.
- **Footwear:** Comfortable shoes for walking or hiking, plus sandals or slip-ons for casual wear.
- **Reusable water bottle:** Many retreats promote sustainability, so carrying a refillable water bottle is both practical and eco-friendly.
- **Journal:** A retreat is a deeply reflective time, and journaling can help you process your experiences and personal growth.
- **Sunscreen and natural bug repellent:** If your retreat is outdoors, protect yourself from the sun and insects with natural, eco-friendly products.
- **Personal wellness items:** Bring along any personal items that enhance your wellness routine, such as essential oils, crystals, or your yoga mat (if the retreat doesn't provide one).

Conclusion

As we come to the end of our journey through the world of wellness retreats, it's important to reflect on how these experiences can shape not just the way you travel, but also the way you live. 2025 is the perfect year to embark on new adventures, whether you're seeking rejuvenation, personal growth, or simply a break from the chaos of daily life.

Embracing Wellness as a Lifelong Journey

A wellness retreat is not just a temporary escape but can be the start of a lifelong commitment to health and well-being. While the retreats themselves offer structured programs, expert guidance, and serene environments, the real challenge is taking what you learn and integrating it into your everyday routine.

The mind-body practices, nutritional habits, and mental clarity you experience at a retreat don't have to be left behind when you board your flight home. In fact, one of the greatest gifts a wellness retreat offers is the ability to take these tools with you—mindfulness exercises, meditation techniques, yoga sequences, or even meal planning approaches can all be adapted into daily rituals.

Practical Tip: Start small. If you fell in love with the meditation sessions, begin incorporating just 5-10 minutes of mindfulness into your morning routine. Similarly, if you discovered a newfound passion for yoga, commit to a couple of online classes each week.

Setting Intentions for the New Year

One of the central themes of wellness retreats is the idea of setting intentions. As you look ahead to the rest of 2025, ask yourself: What do you want to achieve, both personally and in terms of your wellness? Whether it's better mental clarity, improved physical health, or enhanced emotional resilience, identifying your goals is a crucial step.

Consider how the lessons you've learned throughout your retreat experience can contribute to these goals. Maybe you've discovered a passion for mindful eating or a love for nature-based wellness practices. Whatever it is, setting clear and actionable intentions will help you move forward with purpose.

Practical Tip: Write down your top three wellness goals for 2025. Keep them somewhere visible—on your desk, your fridge, or your phone background. Regularly check in on your progress and adjust where needed.

Making Wellness a Part of Your Travel Routine

Wellness retreats aren't the only way to enjoy a mindful, healthy journey. The principles of wellness travel can be applied to any trip, whether you're off on a weekend city break or a long-haul adventure. Prioritize balance in your itinerary by scheduling time for relaxation and reflection, in addition to sightseeing or activities.

Simple adjustments can turn any vacation into a wellness-focused escape. For example, you can practice mindfulness by staying present during a hike, or you can opt for healthy, locally-sourced meals to nourish your body while exploring new cuisines.

Practical Tip: Consider incorporating mini-wellness activities into your future travel plans. Book a local massage, visit a nature reserve, or start your day with a gentle yoga practice before diving into your planned activities.

Staying Connected to Nature and Your Inner Self

Many retreats focus on reconnecting with nature, an element of wellness that is incredibly healing. Whether through forest bathing in Japan, meditative walks in the mountains of Peru, or beach yoga in Bali, nature provides us with a sanctuary for peace and self-discovery.

As you return to your regular life, try to continue this connection with nature. Even if you live in a bustling city, seek out green spaces, parks, or bodies of water where you can find tranquility. Nature not only soothes the mind but also encourages you to stay grounded and mindful of your surroundings.

Practical Tip: Plan weekly "nature breaks"—a walk in a nearby park, a weekend hike, or a few hours spent reading by the beach or lake. Use these moments to disconnect from screens and reconnect with your inner self.

Post-Retreat Reflection: What Worked and What Didn't?

After attending a retreat, it's crucial to reflect on what worked for you and what didn't. Not every element of a retreat will resonate deeply, and that's okay. Perhaps you found the detox diet too restrictive, but loved the meditation workshops. Maybe you enjoyed the group dynamics but realized you prefer solo activities for reflection.

Taking time to reflect allows you to fine-tune your personal wellness routine. Pay attention to what practices you're genuinely excited to incorporate into your life.

Practical Tip: Keep a wellness journal post-retreat. Record your thoughts about your experience, highlighting what you enjoyed and what you'd change. Use this journal to track how you implement new wellness practices in your daily life.

Looking Forward: Planning Your Next Adventure

Wellness is a journey, not a destination. As 2025 unfolds, consider planning future wellness escapes, whether they are week-long retreats or simple weekend getaways that recharge you. The beauty of wellness travel is that there are endless options available, tailored to your evolving needs.

Your wellness journey might lead you to different destinations—a retreat in a new country, or even a revisit to a place that felt like home. Take the time to research and find what excites you, keeping in mind the trends and locations discussed in this guide.

Practical Tip: Bookmark wellness retreat platforms and websites, and subscribe to newsletters to stay updated on new retreat offerings and special deals. Planning ahead will help you discover new experiences that align with your wellness goals.

Final Words: A Year of Growth and Transformation

2025 is a year filled with potential for personal growth, healing, and adventure. By prioritizing wellness in your travels, you not only nurture your mind, body, and spirit but also create lasting memories and habits that will benefit you for years to come.

Whether you choose to explore wellness retreats across the globe or simply incorporate mindful practices into your everyday life, remember that this journey is unique to you. Be open to new experiences, embrace challenges, and most importantly, enjoy the adventure.

Practical Tip: As you look back on the year, celebrate your achievements, no matter how small. Whether it's a new wellness practice, a healthy habit, or a personal milestone, recognize your progress and use it as motivation for the years to come.